Multiple Sclerosis Remission

Secret Strategies for Thriving with Multiple Sclerosis

BY

Dr. Luna Jefferson

Copyright

No part of this book should be copied, reproduced

without the author's permission © 2023

TABLE OF CONTENT

INTRODUCTION 5

   The Central Nervous SystemThe Central Nervous System 6

   Autoimmune Nature of Multiple Sclerosis (MS).....................7

CHAPTER ONE...8

Who Is at Risk? 9

   Demographics and Statistics..10

   Genetic and Environmental Factors 11

   Lifestyle and Controllable Risk Factors 13

CHAPTER TWO...14

Types of Multiple Sclerosis..14

   Relapsing-Remitting MS (RRMS)....................................16

   Secondary Progressive Multiple Sclerosis (SPMS) 18

   Primary Progressive Multiple Sclerosis (PPMS) 19

   Variations and Progression..20

CHAPTER THREE 21

Diagnosing Multiple Sclerosis...22

   The Diagnostic Process 24

   Medical Examinations and Tests 25

   Common Symptoms 27

CHAPTER FOUR 29

Impact on Daily Life...30

   Physical Challenges...32

   Emotional and Social Aspects 34

CHAPTER FIVE..36

Medical Treatments 36

   Disease-Modifying Medications 38

   Importance of Early Intervention 40

   Managing Symptoms 42

CHAPTER SIX...44

Lifestyle Changes...44

   Diet and Nutrition...46

Exercise and Mobility 48

Stress Management..50

CHAPTER SEVEN 53

Nutrition and Multiple sclerosis...53

The Role of Nutrition 55

A Well-Balanced Diet...57

Dietary Considerations 59

CHAPTER EIGHT 61

Specific Diets 61

Mediterranean Diet...63

Low-Fat Diets 65

High-Vitamin D Diets 66

CHAPTER NINE...70

Supplements 70

Vitamin D and MS...72

Omega-3 Fatty Acids..74

Consultation with Healthcare Professionals..................75

CHAPTER TEN 77

Preventive Measures...78

Lifestyle Choices 80

Emerging Research on Prevention 81

CHAPTER ELEVEN 83

Research and Future Therapies..84

Ongoing Research..86

Emerging Therapies..88

Hope for the Future...90

CHAPTER TWELVE 91

Support Networks 92

Importance of Support 94

Community Resources..96

Building a Supportive Network...98

Conclusion 100

Summary of Key Points..101

Encouragement and Empowerment 103

INTRODUCTION

Understanding Multiple Sclerosis (MS) is a journey into the intricate workings of the central nervous system and the challenges faced by those grappling with this autoimmune disorder. At its core, MS involves the immune system mistakenly attacking the protective myelin sheath around nerve fibers, disrupting the smooth communication between the brain and the body. This disruption manifests in a myriad of symptoms, ranging from fatigue and numbness to difficulties with coordination and vision.

The central nervous system, comprising the brain and spinal cord, plays a pivotal role in controlling bodily functions. In MS, the immune system's assault on myelin leads to the formation of scar tissue (sclerosis), hindering the transmission of electrical impulses. The result is a diverse array of symptoms that vary in severity and duration, creating a complex and often unpredictable landscape for those affected.

Understanding MS involves unraveling the genetic and environmental factors that contribute to its onset, delving into the distinct types of the disease, and appreciating the impact it can have on daily life. This comprehension serves as a foundation for exploring effective management strategies, the latest medical treatments, and the ongoing quest for a deeper understanding that fuels hope for the future.

The Central Nervous SystemThe Central Nervous System

The central nervous system (CNS) stands as the intricate command center of the human body, orchestrating and regulating vital functions. Comprising the brain and spinal cord, the CNS is a marvel of biological engineering, responsible for interpreting sensory information, coordinating motor responses, and governing cognitive processes.

At the core of this complex network is the brain, an organ of unparalleled complexity. Divided into regions with specialized functions, the brain processes information, stores memories, and governs emotions. It acts as the epicenter for conscious thought and voluntary actions, making it the seat of human identity.

Connected to the brain is the spinal cord, a long, slender bundle of nerves that extends from the base of the brain down the vertebral column. The spinal cord serves as a conduit for communication between the brain and the rest of the body, facilitating the transmission of electrical signals that govern movement and sensation.

Together, the brain and spinal cord form an integrated system that controls every aspect of our being. The CNS not only responds to external stimuli but also plays a crucial role in maintaining internal balance, ensuring the body functions harmoniously. Understanding the central nervous system is fundamental to comprehending various neurological conditions, including disorders like multiple sclerosis, where disruptions in this intricate system can have profound effects on health and well-being.

Autoimmune Nature of Multiple Sclerosis (MS)

Multiple Sclerosis (MS) is distinguished by its autoimmune nature, marking a condition where the body's immune system turns against its own tissues. In the case of MS, this immune misdirection targets the central nervous system (CNS), specifically the myelin sheath—a protective covering surrounding nerve fibers. The myelin sheath is crucial for the smooth transmission of electrical impulses, facilitating efficient communication between the brain and the rest of the body.

In MS, immune cells mistakenly identify the myelin as a threat and launch an attack, triggering inflammation and causing damage to the myelin. This immune assault leads to the formation of scar tissue, or sclerosis, disrupting the normal flow of electrical signals. As a consequence, individuals with MS experience a spectrum of neurological symptoms, ranging from numbness and tingling to more severe challenges like impaired mobility and vision issues.

Understanding the autoimmune nature of MS is paramount for both patients and researchers alike. It prompts exploration into the factors triggering this immune response, delving into genetic predispositions and environmental influences. Unraveling the intricacies of the autoimmune component is a crucial step toward developing targeted therapies that may modulate or mitigate the immune response, ultimately offering hope for more effective treatments and improved quality of life for those affected by MS.

CHAPTER ONE

Who Is at Risk?

Identifying who is at risk for Multiple Sclerosis (MS) involves navigating a complex interplay of genetic, environmental, and demographic factors. While the exact cause remains elusive, certain trends have emerged, shedding light on populations more susceptible to this autoimmune disorder. Research suggests a higher risk for individuals with a family history of MS, indicating a genetic predisposition that may contribute to susceptibility.

Geographical location plays a role, with higher prevalence observed in regions farther from the equator. This geographic pattern implies a potential link to sunlight exposure and vitamin D levels, though the precise connection is still under exploration. Gender is another factor, as MS disproportionately affects women more than men.

Environmental elements such as viral infections, particularly during childhood, have been implicated in triggering MS in genetically susceptible individuals. Additionally, lifestyle factors like smoking and obesity may elevate the risk of developing the disease.

While these risk factors provide insights, it's important to note that MS can affect individuals without these characteristics. The interplay of genetics and environment remains complex, and ongoing research strives to unravel the intricacies of who is at risk and why. Understanding these risk factors is crucial for early intervention, monitoring, and developing preventive strategies to reduce the impact of MS on vulnerable populations.

Demographics and Statistics

Demographics and statistics paint a nuanced picture of the prevalence and impact of Multiple Sclerosis (MS) across diverse populations. MS, a neurological autoimmune disorder, exhibits demographic patterns that highlight its complex nature. Globally, it is estimated that around 2.8 million people are living with MS, with varying prevalence rates in different regions.

One notable demographic trend is the higher incidence of MS in women compared to men, with women being two to three times more likely to develop the condition. The onset of MS typically occurs between the ages of 20 and 50, although cases can emerge at any age. Moreover, MS displays a geographical gradient, with higher prevalence rates observed in regions farther from the equator, suggesting a potential link between sunlight exposure, vitamin D, and the development of the disease.

Certain ethnic backgrounds, such as those of Northern European descent, have a higher risk of MS, while individuals of African, Asian, and Native American descent generally have lower risk rates. These demographic patterns underscore the interplay of genetic and environmental factors in MS susceptibility.

Understanding the demographics of MS is crucial for healthcare planning, resource allocation, and developing targeted interventions. As research continues, these demographic insights contribute to a more comprehensive understanding of the disease and aid in tailoring approaches to address its diverse impact on individuals and communities.

Genetic and Environmental Factors

Multiple Sclerosis (MS) is a multifaceted condition influenced by a delicate interplay of genetic and environmental factors. The role of genetics in MS is evident through familial patterns, where individuals with a family history of the disease have an increased risk. Specific genes associated with immune system regulation and responses may contribute to susceptibility, highlighting the hereditary component.

Environmental factors also play a pivotal role in the development of MS. Exposure to certain viruses, particularly during childhood, has been implicated as a potential trigger. Additionally, there is a notable correlation between geographical location and MS prevalence, with higher rates observed in regions farther from the equator. This geographical pattern suggests a link between sunlight exposure, vitamin D levels, and the risk of developing MS.

Furthermore, lifestyle choices such as smoking and obesity are environmental factors that may heighten susceptibility to MS. Smoking, in particular, has been identified as a significant risk factor, exacerbating the impact of the disease.

Understanding the intricate dance between genetic predisposition and environmental influences is crucial in unraveling the mysteries of MS. Ongoing research aims to dissect these factors further, shedding light on the mechanisms that initiate and perpetuate the autoimmune response, ultimately paving the way for targeted prevention strategies and more effective treatments.

Lifestyle and Controllable Risk Factors

Lifestyle choices and controllable risk factors play a pivotal role in the management and prevention of Multiple Sclerosis (MS). While the underlying causes of MS remain complex, certain lifestyle modifications can positively impact the course of the disease and potentially reduce the risk of onset.

Maintaining a healthy and balanced diet is a cornerstone of managing MS. Adopting an anti-inflammatory diet rich in fruits, vegetables, and omega-3 fatty acids can contribute to overall well-being. Studies suggest that a diet low in saturated fats and high in vitamin D may have a protective effect.

Regular physical activity is another controllable factor that influences the progression of MS. Exercise not only helps in maintaining mobility and strength but also contributes to improved mood and overall quality of life for individuals with MS.

Stress management is crucial, as stress can exacerbate MS symptoms. Techniques such as mindfulness, meditation, and yoga can be valuable tools in mitigating stress and promoting mental well-being.

Avoiding tobacco smoke is imperative, as smoking has been linked to an increased risk of developing MS and can worsen the course of the disease. Additionally, maintaining a healthy weight and avoiding excessive alcohol consumption are factors that can positively impact the overall health of individuals with or at risk for MS.

Empowering individuals with knowledge about controllable risk factors allows them to take an active role in managing their health and well-being in the face of this complex neurological condition.

CHAPTER TWO

Types of Multiple Sclerosis

Multiple Sclerosis (MS) manifests in several distinct types, each with its characteristic course and progression. Understanding these types is crucial for tailoring treatment plans and managing the diverse challenges posed by the disease.

1. Relapsing-Remitting MS (RRMS):
   - This is the most common form of MS, characterized by clearly defined relapses or exacerbations of symptoms followed by periods of partial or complete recovery. Between relapses, individuals often experience periods of stability.

2. Secondary Progressive MS (SPMS):
   - After a period of relapsing-remitting disease, some individuals may transition to secondary progressive MS, where symptoms gradually worsen over time with or

without distinct relapses. SPMS may still involve periods of stability or temporary improvement.

3. Primary Progressive MS (PPMS):
  - PPMS is characterized by a steady worsening of symptoms from the onset, without distinct relapses. This form is less common but tends to be associated with more rapid disability progression.

4. Progressive-Relapsing MS (PRMS):
  - A less common subtype, PRMS involves a steady worsening of symptoms with occasional relapses and periods of stability. Disability accumulates over time, distinguishing it from relapsing-remitting forms.

5. Clinically Isolated Syndrome (CIS):
  - CIS is not a type of Multiple sclerosis but a single episode of neurological symptoms lasting at least 24 hours. However, it is considered significant because it may precede a diagnosis of MS, particularly if accompanied by specific MRI findings.

The diversity of MS types underscores the complexity of the disease, making individualized treatment and management crucial. Advances in research and treatment options continue to refine our understanding of these different types, offering hope for improved outcomes and quality of life for those affected by Multiple sclerosis.

Relapsing-Remitting MS (RRMS)

Relapsing-Remitting Multiple Sclerosis (RRMS) is the most prevalent and well-recognized form of this autoimmune neurological disorder. Characterized by distinct episodes of symptom exacerbation, known as relapses or flare-ups, followed by periods of partial or complete recovery, RRMS presents a cyclical pattern of disease activity.

During a relapse, individuals with RRMS may experience a sudden onset or worsening of neurological symptoms, such as fatigue, numbness, impaired coordination, or vision problems. These episodes can vary in duration and intensity. Following a relapse, there is a period of remission, during which symptoms stabilize or improve, allowing individuals to regain some function and resume daily activities.

The unpredictable nature of RRMS poses challenges for those living with the condition, as the frequency and severity of relapses can vary widely. Despite the episodic nature of the disease, RRMS may eventually transition into a secondary progressive phase, marked by a gradual accumulation of disability over time.

Treatment strategies for RRMS often involve disease-modifying therapies aimed at reducing the frequency and severity of relapses, slowing disease progression, and managing symptoms. The management of RRMS requires a personalized approach, considering the unique experiences and needs of each individual, emphasizing the importance of ongoing medical monitoring and adaptation of treatment plans.

Secondary Progressive Multiple Sclerosis (SPMS)

Secondary Progressive Multiple Sclerosis (SPMS) represents a phase in the continuum of this complex neurological disorder, typically following an initial period of Relapsing-Remitting MS (RRMS). In SPMS, individuals experience a gradual and sustained worsening of neurological function, marked by a progressive accumulation of disability over time.

Unlike RRMS, SPMS is characterized by a more steady decline in health without distinct relapses. The transition from RRMS to SPMS varies among individuals, with some experiencing a gradual shift, while others may notice a more abrupt onset of progressive symptoms.

This phase often begins after several years of living with RRMS, typically in mid-to-late adulthood.

Managing SPMS poses unique challenges, and treatment strategies aim to alleviate symptoms, improve quality of life, and slow the progression of disability. Disease-modifying therapies that have demonstrated efficacy in RRMS may be considered, and symptomatic treatments play a crucial role in addressing specific challenges associated with SPMS.

The unpredictable nature of SPMS underscores the importance of ongoing medical evaluation and personalized care plans. Research continues to explore novel therapies and interventions that may offer hope for slowing the progression of disability in individuals navigating the complexities of Secondary Progressive MS.

Primary Progressive Multiple Sclerosis (PPMS)

Primary Progressive Multiple Sclerosis (PPMS) stands as a less common but distinctive form of this chronic autoimmune disorder affecting the central nervous system. Unlike Relapsing-Remitting MS, PPMS is characterized by a steady and continuous worsening of symptoms from the onset, without distinct periods of relapse and remission.

Individuals with PPMS typically experience a gradual accumulation of disability, often involving difficulties with mobility, balance, and coordination. The onset of PPMS commonly occurs in the later stages of adulthood, and the progression of disability can vary widely among individuals.

Managing PPMS presents unique challenges as there are currently limited treatment options specifically approved for this form of MS. Symptomatic treatments and rehabilitation strategies, including physical and occupational therapy, play a crucial role in enhancing quality of life and maintaining functional independence.

Research into the underlying mechanisms of PPMS and the development of targeted therapies are ongoing, offering hope for improved outcomes and a better understanding of this particular manifestation of MS. The journey with Primary Progressive MS emphasizes the importance of personalized care plans, adaptive strategies, and ongoing support for individuals facing the continuous progression of symptoms.

Variations and Progression

The variations in the presentation and progression of Multiple Sclerosis (MS) underscore the complexity of this neurological disorder. MS is often described as a heterogeneous condition due to the diverse ways it can manifest and progress in different individuals.

Variations in MS extend beyond the well-known subtypes (Relapsing-Remitting, Secondary Progressive, Primary Progressive) to include a spectrum of symptom combinations and severity levels. The range of neurological symptoms—such as fatigue, cognitive impairment, numbness, and motor dysfunction—can vary widely, making each individual's experience unique.

Progression of MS is equally variable. While some individuals may experience relatively stable periods, others may face a more continuous decline in neurological function. Factors influencing progression include the type of MS, genetics, lifestyle, and the efficacy of treatment strategies.

Understanding the myriad ways MS can present and progress is essential for both healthcare providers and individuals living with the condition. Personalized treatment plans, adapted to the specific needs and challenges of each person, become paramount in managing this complex and unpredictable disease. Ongoing research aimed at unraveling the intricate factors contributing to these variations holds promise for refining treatment approaches and improving the overall quality of life for those navigating the diverse landscape of Multiple Sclerosis.

CHAPTER THREE

Diagnosing Multiple Sclerosis

Diagnosing Multiple Sclerosis (MS) is a nuanced process that involves a comprehensive evaluation of clinical symptoms, medical history, and diagnostic tests. No single test can definitively confirm the presence of MS, making the diagnostic journey intricate and often requiring collaboration between neurologists and other healthcare professionals.

1. Medical History and Clinical Evaluation:
   - The diagnostic process typically begins with a detailed medical history to understand the onset, duration, and nature of symptoms. A thorough neurological examination assesses functions such as coordination, reflexes, and sensory perception.

2. Magnetic Resonance Imaging (MRI):

- MRI scans of the brain and spinal cord are crucial for visualizing the presence of lesions or areas of demyelination. These images help confirm the spatial and temporal dissemination of lesions, a key criterion for an MS diagnosis.

3. Cerebrospinal Fluid Analysis:
   - Lumbar puncture or spinal tap may be performed to analyze the cerebrospinal fluid for the presence of immune system markers and antibodies, providing additional evidence of central nervous system inflammation.

4. Evoked Potential Tests:
   - These tests measure the electrical activity in response to stimuli, such as visual or auditory stimuli, helping identify delays in nerve signal transmission.

5. Blood Tests:
   - Blood tests are conducted to rule out other conditions that may mimic MS symptoms and to assess specific biomarkers associated with the disease.

Diagnosing MS is often a process of exclusion, ruling out other potential causes of symptoms. The complexity of this process highlights the importance of a skilled and experienced medical team working collaboratively to provide an accurate diagnosis and initiate appropriate treatment strategies tailored to the individual's unique circumstances.

The Diagnostic Process

The diagnostic process for Multiple Sclerosis (MS) is a meticulous journey that involves a combination of clinical assessments, advanced imaging techniques, and laboratory tests. This process is essential for distinguishing MS from other conditions with similar symptoms and confirming the presence of demyelination in the central nervous system.

1. Medical History and Clinical Examination:
   - A thorough review of the patient's medical history, including the onset and progression of symptoms, is the starting point. Neurologists conduct a comprehensive clinical examination to evaluate motor function, sensory perception, coordination, and reflexes.

2. Magnetic Resonance Imaging (MRI):
   - MRI scans of the brain and spinal cord are pivotal. Lesions or areas of demyelination appear as distinctive white spots on these images. The location and dissemination of these lesions over time contribute to the diagnostic criteria for MS.

3. Cerebrospinal Fluid Analysis:
  - A lumbar puncture may be performed to analyze cerebrospinal fluid for the presence of immune system markers and antibodies. Elevated levels of certain proteins can support the diagnosis of MS.

4. Evoked Potential Tests:
  - These tests measure the electrical activity in response to stimuli and can reveal delays in nerve signal transmission, providing additional evidence of central nervous system involvement.

5. Blood Tests:
  - Blood tests help rule out other conditions that may mimic MS symptoms and assess specific biomarkers associated with the disease.

The diagnostic process is often iterative, requiring collaboration between neurologists, radiologists, and other specialists. While there is no single definitive test for MS, the combination of these diagnostic tools helps establish a comprehensive understanding of the individual's condition, enabling the development of tailored treatment plans.

Medical Examinations and Tests

Medical examinations and tests play a pivotal role in the diagnostic journey for Multiple Sclerosis (MS), helping healthcare professionals unravel the complexities of this neurological disorder. These assessments are crucial for confirming the presence of demyelination, determining the type of MS, and ruling out other conditions with similar symptoms.

1. Neurological Examination:
   - A thorough neurological examination involves evaluating sensory functions, motor skills, reflexes, coordination, and cognitive abilities. Neurologists carefully assess symptoms and their impact on daily life.

2. Magnetic Resonance Imaging (MRI):
   - MRI scans provide detailed images of the brain and spinal cord, revealing the presence, location, and dissemination of lesions or areas of demyelination. This imaging technique is a cornerstone in diagnosing and monitoring MS.

3. Cerebrospinal Fluid Analysis:
   - A lumbar puncture, or spinal tap, allows the collection and analysis of cerebrospinal fluid. Elevated levels of certain proteins and the presence of oligoclonal

bands can provide evidence of inflammation in the central nervous system.

4. Evoked Potential Tests:
   - These tests measure the electrical activity in response to stimuli, such as visual or auditory cues, detecting delays in nerve signal transmission that may indicate demyelination.

5. Blood Tests:
   - Blood tests help rule out other conditions that may mimic MS symptoms and assess specific biomarkers associated with the disease.

By combining information from these medical examinations and tests, healthcare professionals can establish a comprehensive understanding of the individual's condition, guiding the diagnostic process and informing tailored treatment strategies for managing the complexities of Multiple Sclerosis.

Common Symptoms

Multiple Sclerosis (MS) manifests with a diverse array of symptoms, varying in severity and duration. These symptoms arise from the disruption of nerve signals due to inflammation, demyelination, and, in advanced stages, nerve damage. Common symptoms of MS span various aspects of neurological function and can profoundly impact daily life.

1. Fatigue:
 - Overwhelming fatigue is a pervasive symptom in MS, often unrelated to physical exertion. It can significantly affect daily activities and quality of life.

2. Numbness and Tingling:
 - Sensory disturbances, such as numbness, tingling, or a "pins and needles" sensation, often occur, affecting different parts of the body.

3. Motor Dysfunction:
 - Weakness, muscle stiffness, and difficulty with coordination and balance can hinder mobility, leading to challenges in walking and performing fine motor tasks.

4. Vision Problems:
 - Optic neuritis is a common symptom, causing blurred vision, eye pain, and sometimes a temporary loss of vision.

5. Cognitive Impairment:
 - Memory lapses, difficulty concentrating, and other cognitive challenges can affect information processing and daily cognitive tasks.

6. Bladder and Bowel Dysfunction:
   - MS can disrupt nerve signals controlling bladder and bowel function, resulting in issues such as incontinence or difficulty emptying the bladder.

7. Spasticity and Pain:
   - Muscle stiffness and spasms are frequent, often accompanied by neuropathic pain that can be localized or widespread.

8. Emotional and Psychological Changes:
   - Mood swings, depression, and anxiety are common, potentially influenced by the neurological and emotional impact of the condition.

Understanding the breadth of these common symptoms is crucial for both individuals with MS and healthcare providers, as it informs comprehensive management strategies tailored to address the unique challenges faced by each person navigating the complexities of this chronic neurological condition.

CHAPTER FOUR

Impact on Daily Life

The impact of Multiple Sclerosis (MS) on daily life is profound and multifaceted, as this chronic neurological condition can affect various aspects of physical, emotional, and social well-being. Individuals with MS often grapple with a range of challenges that necessitate adaptive strategies and resilience.

1. Mobility and Independence:
 - Progressive weakness, muscle stiffness, and impaired coordination can significantly affect mobility. Tasks like walking, climbing stairs, or even performing routine activities become challenging, requiring the use of mobility aids or assistive devices.

2. Fatigue and Energy Levels:
 - Persistent fatigue is a pervasive symptom in MS, leading to decreased energy levels. This fatigue can limit the ability to engage in activities and necessitate

strategic planning to conserve energy throughout the day.

3. Cognitive Function:

  - Cognitive symptoms, including difficulties with memory, concentration, and problem-solving, impact daily cognitive tasks. Individuals may find it challenging to manage work responsibilities, household tasks, and other cognitive demands.

4. Emotional Well-being:

  - The unpredictable nature of MS, coupled with the physical and cognitive challenges, can contribute to emotional struggles. Depression, anxiety, and mood swings are common, highlighting the need for emotional support and mental health care.

5. Social Interactions:

  - MS can influence social interactions as individuals may experience limitations in participating in social events or face challenges related to mobility and fatigue. Maintaining social connections becomes crucial for emotional well-being.

6. Occupational Impact:

  - The ability to work may be compromised due to physical limitations or cognitive difficulties. Adaptations, such as flexible work schedules or modifications to the work environment, may be necessary.

7. Daily Activities:

- Simple daily activities, such as dressing, grooming, and preparing meals, may require creative solutions and adaptive equipment to overcome physical limitations.

Navigating the impact of MS on daily life necessitates a holistic and individualized approach. Rehabilitation, assistive technologies, emotional support, and lifestyle adjustments are integral components of managing the challenges posed by MS, empowering individuals to maintain independence and enhance their overall quality of life.

Physical Challenges

The physical challenges posed by Multiple Sclerosis (MS) are diverse and often profound, affecting various aspects of mobility, coordination, and overall physical well-being. These challenges stem from the damage to the central nervous system, disrupting the transmission of signals between the brain and the rest of the body.

1. Mobility Limitations:

- Progressive weakness and muscle stiffness can result in difficulties with walking and coordination. Many individuals with MS may require mobility aids like canes, walkers, or wheelchairs to maintain independence.

2. Spasticity and Muscle Spasms:
  - Spasticity, characterized by muscle tightness and involuntary spasms, is a common symptom. These spasms can be painful and hinder smooth, controlled movements.

3. Balance and Coordination Issues:
  - Impaired balance and coordination are frequent challenges, increasing the risk of falls. Activities that involve precise movements, such as reaching for objects or navigating stairs, become more difficult.

4. Fine Motor Skill Impairments:
  - Deterioration in fine motor skills can impact everyday tasks like buttoning clothes, writing, or using utensils. Adaptive tools and strategies may be necessary.

5. Fatigue:
  - Debilitating fatigue is a pervasive physical challenge in MS, often unrelated to exertion. It can exacerbate other symptoms and limit the ability to engage in daily activities.

6. Bladder and Bowel Dysfunction:

- Disruption of nerve signals controlling bladder and bowel function can lead to incontinence or difficulties with elimination, posing additional physical challenges.

Addressing these physical challenges involves a multidisciplinary approach, including physical therapy, rehabilitation, and the use of assistive devices. Individualized strategies are crucial to enhancing mobility, minimizing discomfort, and optimizing overall physical function for individuals navigating the complexities of living with MS.

Emotional and Social Aspects

The emotional and social aspects of living with Multiple Sclerosis (MS) are integral components of the overall impact of this chronic neurological condition. MS not only poses physical challenges but also engenders a range of emotions and influences social interactions, requiring resilience and support.

1. Emotional Impact:
- The unpredictability of MS, coupled with the physical limitations it imposes, can give rise to a spectrum of emotions. Individuals may grapple with fear, anxiety, frustration, and grief over the perceived loss of abilities.

Coping with the chronic nature of the disease requires ongoing emotional resilience.

2. Depression and Anxiety:
   - The chronic nature of MS, coupled with the potential for disability progression, can contribute to mental health challenges. Depression and anxiety are common, necessitating both emotional support and professional mental health care.

3. Social Isolation:
   - Physical limitations, fatigue, and the unpredictable nature of symptoms can lead to social isolation. Individuals with MS may face challenges participating in social events, maintaining regular social connections, or engaging in activities they once enjoyed.

4. Impact on Relationships:
   - MS can influence relationships with family, friends, and romantic partners. Communication and understanding become crucial, as the dynamics of relationships may shift due to the challenges posed by the condition.

5. Work and Career:
   - The impact of MS on career and occupational aspects can contribute to stress and feelings of inadequacy. Navigating workplace challenges and potential adjustments may be emotionally taxing.

Support networks, including friends, family, and MS-specific communities, play a vital role in addressing the emotional and social dimensions of living with MS. Open communication, counseling, and participation in support groups contribute to a holistic approach in enhancing emotional well-being and fostering meaningful social connections.

CHAPTER FIVE

Medical Treatments

Medical treatments for Multiple Sclerosis (MS) aim to manage symptoms, slow disease progression, and improve overall quality of life. The complex nature of MS requires a multidisciplinary approach, and treatment plans are often tailored to individual needs. Several key medical interventions are employed:

1. Disease-Modifying Therapies (DMTs):
   - DMTs are a cornerstone in managing MS, particularly in the relapsing forms. These medications, administered orally or via injection, help modulate the immune system to reduce the frequency and severity of relapses and slow down disease progression.

2. Immunosuppressive Therapies:
   - For individuals with aggressive forms of MS, immunosuppressive therapies may be recommended to dampen the immune response. These treatments are

often reserved for cases where other interventions have not been effective.

3. Corticosteroids:
  - During relapses, corticosteroids such as methylprednisolone may be prescribed to reduce inflammation and shorten the duration of symptoms. These are often administered in short courses.

4. Symptomatic Treatments:
  - Symptomatic treatments address specific MS symptoms. For example, muscle relaxants may be prescribed for spasticity, medications for neuropathic pain, and medications to manage bladder dysfunction.

5. Rehabilitation Therapies:
  - Physical therapy, occupational therapy, and speech therapy are integral components of MS management. These therapies focus on enhancing mobility, maintaining independence, and addressing cognitive challenges.

6. Plasma Exchange (Plasmapheresis):
  - In severe cases or during acute relapses, plasma exchange may be considered to remove antibodies from the blood that are contributing to the immune response.

7. Experimental and Emerging Therapies:

- Ongoing research explores novel treatment approaches, including stem cell therapies and emerging medications, offering hope for more targeted and effective interventions.

Treatment decisions are made collaboratively between individuals with MS and their healthcare team, considering factors such as the type and stage of MS, individual health status, and preferences. Regular monitoring and adjustments to treatment plans are essential to optimize outcomes and improve the overall well-being of those living with Multiple Sclerosis.

Disease-Modifying Medications

Disease-Modifying Medications (DMTs) represent a pivotal category of treatments in the management of Multiple Sclerosis (MS). These medications play a crucial role in altering the course of the disease by modulating the immune system and reducing the frequency and severity of relapses. DMTs are primarily used in the treatment of relapsing forms of MS and have demonstrated efficacy in slowing down the progression of disability.

These medications act on various components of the immune system to prevent or suppress the autoimmune response responsible for attacking the central nervous system. Common types of DMTs include interferons, glatiramer acetate, oral medications like fingolimod and teriflunomide, and newer monoclonal antibodies such as ocrelizumab and natalizumab.

The choice of a specific DMT is often based on individual factors such as the type and severity of MS, potential side effects, and the patient's lifestyle. Regular monitoring, including imaging studies and clinical assessments, helps healthcare professionals evaluate the effectiveness of DMTs and make adjustments as needed. While DMTs do not provide a cure for MS, they significantly contribute to managing the disease, improving quality of life, and slowing down the progression of disability for many individuals living with this complex neurological condition.

Here is a list of some DMTs that were commonly used for MS treatment as of 2022:

- Interferon Beta-1a (Avonex, Rebif)
- Interferon Beta-1b (Betaseron, Extavia)
- Glatiramer Acetate (Copaxone, Glatopa)
- Dimethyl Fumarate (Tecfidera)
- Teriflunomide (Aubagio)
- Fingolimod (Gilenya)

- ◆ Natalizumab (Tysabri)
- ◆ Alemtuzumab (Lemtrada)

Importance of Early Intervention

Early intervention in Multiple Sclerosis (MS) is of paramount importance as it can significantly impact the course of the disease and the quality of life for individuals affected. Timely diagnosis and initiation of appropriate treatments offer several key advantages:

1. Disease Modulation:
   - Early intervention with disease-modifying therapies (DMTs) can help modulate the immune system, reducing the frequency and severity of relapses. This, in turn, may slow down the progression of disability and potentially preserve neurological function.

2. Prevention of Accumulated Damage:
   - By addressing inflammation and demyelination early on, interventions may prevent the accumulation of irreversible damage to the central nervous system. Protecting nerve fibers from sustained injury can lead to better long-term outcomes.

3. Improved Symptom Management:

- Early identification allows for prompt management of symptoms, addressing issues such as fatigue, pain, and mobility challenges more effectively. Symptomatic treatments and rehabilitation strategies can be implemented early to enhance overall well-being.

4. Enhanced Quality of Life:

- Early intervention supports individuals in maintaining a higher quality of life by minimizing the impact of the disease on daily activities, relationships, and occupational pursuits. This is particularly crucial in preserving independence and functional abilities.

5. Optimized Treatment Plans:

- Early diagnosis provides a window of opportunity for healthcare professionals to tailor treatment plans based on individual characteristics and preferences, optimizing the overall approach to MS management.

The evolving landscape of MS research underscores the importance of early intervention in shaping more effective and personalized treatment strategies. Encouraging awareness, regular healthcare check-ups, and proactive engagement with healthcare providers facilitate early detection and intervention, offering individuals with MS the best possible prospects for a more favorable disease trajectory.

Managing Symptoms

Managing the complications of Multiple Sclerosis (MS) requires a comprehensive and multidisciplinary approach, addressing both the physical and emotional aspects of the condition. While MS manifests differently in individuals, common complications include mobility issues, fatigue, cognitive changes, and emotional well-being. Here's a detailed overview of management procedures for these complications:

1. Mobility Issues:
   - *Physical Therapy:* Tailored exercise programs designed by physical therapists can improve strength, balance, and coordination, addressing mobility challenges.
   - *Assistive Devices:* Walking aids, wheelchairs, and other assistive devices enhance independence and safety for individuals with mobility limitations.
   - Adaptive Techniques: Learning adaptive techniques for daily activities can help individuals conserve energy and move more efficiently.

2. Fatigue:
   - *Energy Conservation Strategies:* Balancing activity and rest, prioritizing tasks, and breaking activities into smaller, manageable segments can help manage fatigue.

- ***Physical Activity:*** Regular, low-impact exercise, such as swimming or yoga, can combat fatigue and improve overall energy levels.

- ***Sleep Hygiene:*** Ensuring good sleep quality through consistent sleep routines and addressing sleep disorders contributes to reducing fatigue.

3. Cognitive Changes:

- ***Cognitive Rehabilitation:*** Cognitive therapy programs and exercises aim to improve memory, attention, and problem-solving skills.

- ***Mental Stimulation:*** Engaging in mentally stimulating activities, such as puzzles or reading, supports cognitive function.

- ***Medication:*** In some cases, medications may be prescribed to manage specific cognitive symptoms.

4. Emotional Well-being:

- ***Counseling and Psychotherapy:*** Mental health professionals can provide support and coping strategies for emotional challenges associated with MS.

- ***Support Groups:*** Joining MS support groups, either in-person or online, fosters a sense of community and understanding.

- ***Mindfulness and Stress Management:*** Techniques such as mindfulness meditation and stress management strategies contribute to emotional well-being.

5. Pain Management:

  - *Medications:* Analgesics and anti-inflammatory medications may be prescribed to manage pain.
  - *Physical Therapy:* Techniques such as massage and stretching, guided by physical therapists, can alleviate pain associated with muscle stiffness or spasms.
  - *Heat and Cold Therapy:* Applying heat or cold to affected areas can provide relief from pain and discomfort.

6. Bladder and Bowel Dysfunction:

  - *Bladder Training:* Timed voiding and fluid management help regulate bladder function.
  - *Pelvic Floor Exercises:* Strengthening pelvic floor muscles through exercises can aid in managing bladder and bowel dysfunction.
  - *Medication:* Certain medications may be prescribed to address specific bladder or bowel issues.

7. Vision Problems:

  - *Optical Devices:* Glasses, contact lenses, or magnifiers can assist with vision issues.
  - *Visual Rehabilitation:* Programs focusing on enhancing visual skills may be recommended for individuals with vision challenges.
  - *Medication:* Some medications can help manage specific visual symptoms.

8. Speech and Swallowing Difficulties:

 - *Speech Therapy:* Speech therapists can provide exercises and techniques to improve speech and swallowing function.
 - *Dietary Modifications:* Adjusting food textures and using specific swallowing techniques may be recommended.
 - *Assistive Devices:* Devices like communication boards can aid individuals with speech difficulties.

It's crucial for individuals with MS to work closely with a healthcare team, including neurologists, physical therapists, occupational therapists, psychologists, and other specialists. A tailored and collaborative approach ensures that management procedures are personalized to address the unique needs and challenges of each individual. Regular communication, ongoing evaluation, and adjustments to the management plan contribute to optimizing overall well-being for those living with MS.

Managing symptoms is a critical aspect of enhancing the quality of life for individuals living with Multiple Sclerosis (MS). Given the diverse range of symptoms that can accompany this neurological condition, a comprehensive and individualized approach is essential for effective symptom management.

1. Pharmacological Interventions:
 - Medications play a key role in symptom management. For example, muscle relaxants can alleviate spasticity,

while pain medications address neuropathic pain. Antidepressants and anti-anxiety medications may help manage emotional symptoms.

2. Physical and Occupational Therapy:
   - Rehabilitation therapies, including physical and occupational therapy, are invaluable for addressing mobility challenges and enhancing independence. These therapies focus on exercises, adaptive strategies, and assistive devices to optimize physical function.

3. Counseling and Psychological Support:
   - Emotional symptoms such as depression and anxiety are common in MS. Counseling and psychological support, including cognitive-behavioral therapy, can provide coping mechanisms and improve mental well-being.

4. Assistive Technologies:
   - Technological aids, such as mobility devices, communication tools, and home modifications, can significantly improve daily functioning. These assistive technologies are tailored to individual needs, promoting autonomy.

5. Lifestyle Modifications:
   - Adopting a healthy lifestyle, including regular exercise, a balanced diet, and stress management, can contribute

to overall well-being. These lifestyle modifications may help alleviate fatigue and improve energy levels.

6. Temperature Management:
  - MS symptoms can be sensitive to temperature changes. Cooling strategies, such as wearing cooling vests or avoiding overheating, can be effective in managing symptoms like fatigue and heat sensitivity.

A collaborative approach involving healthcare professionals, individuals with MS, and their support networks is crucial for successful symptom management. Regular communication, ongoing assessment, and flexibility in adapting strategies to changing needs contribute to a more comprehensive and effective approach to managing the complexities of MS symptoms.

CHAPTER SIX

Lifestyle Changes

Lifestyle changes play a pivotal role in managing Multiple Sclerosis (MS), helping individuals navigate the challenges of this chronic neurological condition and enhance overall well-being. Adopting a holistic approach that encompasses various aspects of daily life can contribute to symptom management and improved quality of life.

1. Dietary Modifications:
   - Embracing a balanced and nutritious diet is crucial for individuals with MS. Some studies suggest that an anti-inflammatory diet, rich in fruits, vegetables, and omega-3 fatty acids, may have potential benefits in managing symptoms.

2. Regular Exercise:
   - Physical activity is beneficial for maintaining mobility, strength, and overall health. Tailored exercise programs,

including aerobic exercises and strength training, can be adapted to individual abilities and preferences.

3. Stress Management:

- Stress can exacerbate MS symptoms. Practices such as mindfulness, meditation, and yoga are effective tools for stress management, promoting relaxation and emotional well-being.

4. Adequate Sleep:

- Prioritizing sufficient and quality sleep is essential. Fatigue is a common symptom of MS, and ensuring proper rest can contribute to improved energy levels and overall health.

5. Smoking Cessation:

- Smoking is a known risk factor for MS progression. Quitting smoking can positively impact the course of the disease and improve overall health.

6. Maintaining a Healthy Weight:

- Achieving and maintaining a healthy weight is important for overall well-being. Obesity can contribute to the progression of MS and exacerbate certain symptoms.

7. Sunlight Exposure:

- Sunlight is a natural source of vitamin D, and adequate levels of vitamin D may have a protective effect in MS. Spending time outdoors and ensuring appropriate sun exposure can contribute to vitamin D synthesis.

Lifestyle changes are most effective when personalized to individual needs and integrated into a comprehensive MS management plan. Consulting with healthcare professionals, including neurologists, dietitians, and rehabilitation specialists, can guide individuals in making informed choices that align with their unique circumstances and health goals.

Diet and Nutrition

Diet and nutrition are integral components of managing Multiple Sclerosis (MS), with emerging evidence suggesting that certain dietary choices may influence symptom management and overall well-being. While there is no specific "MS diet," adopting a healthy and balanced eating plan can have positive effects on various aspects of health for individuals with MS.

1. Anti-Inflammatory Diet:
   - Some research suggests that an anti-inflammatory diet, which includes foods rich in antioxidants, omega-3 fatty acids, and fiber, may be beneficial for individuals with MS. This includes fruits, vegetables, fish, nuts, and whole grains.

2. Vitamin D:

- Adequate levels of vitamin D are crucial for overall health and may have a protective effect in MS. Sun exposure, vitamin D-rich foods (such as fatty fish and fortified dairy products), or supplements can contribute to maintaining optimal levels.

3. Hydration:

- Staying well-hydrated is essential, especially as MS symptoms can be sensitive to dehydration. Opting for water and limiting the intake of sugary beverages supports overall health.

4. Balanced Nutrition:

- Ensuring a well-balanced diet that includes a mix of macronutrients (carbohydrates, proteins, and fats) and micronutrients supports overall health. Individual nutritional needs may vary, and consulting with a registered dietitian can provide personalized guidance.

5. Limiting Saturated Fats:

- Some studies suggest that a diet low in saturated fats may be beneficial for individuals with MS. This involves reducing the intake of red meat, full-fat dairy products, and processed foods high in unhealthy fats.

6. Individualized Approaches:

- Recognizing that each person with MS has unique dietary needs and responses is crucial. What works for one individual may not work for another, and dietary adjustments should be tailored to individual preferences and tolerances.

While research on the specific impact of diet on MS is ongoing, adopting a nutrient-rich, well-balanced diet is generally recommended for overall health. It is essential for individuals with MS to work closely with healthcare professionals, including dietitians, to create an individualized nutrition plan that aligns with their specific health goals and complements their overall MS management strategy.

Exercise and Mobility

Exercise and maintaining mobility are crucial components of managing Multiple Sclerosis (MS), contributing to physical well-being, functional independence, and overall quality of life. While the specific exercise regimen may vary based on individual abilities and symptoms, incorporating regular physical activity has shown several benefits for those with MS.

1. Improved Mobility and Balance:
   - Regular exercise, including both aerobic and strength-training activities, helps enhance muscle strength,

coordination, and balance. This can be particularly beneficial in addressing mobility challenges associated with MS.

2. Fatigue Management:

   - Despite the fatigue often experienced by individuals with MS, appropriate exercise can contribute to increased energy levels and reduced overall fatigue. Tailoring exercise routines to individual capacities is essential to avoid overexertion.

3. Cognitive Benefits:

   - Exercise has been linked to cognitive benefits, which is especially relevant for individuals with MS who may experience cognitive challenges. Engaging in activities that challenge the brain, such as certain forms of aerobic exercise, may support cognitive function.

4. Mood Enhancement:

   - Physical activity is known to release endorphins, promoting a positive mood and reducing symptoms of depression and anxiety, common emotional challenges in MS.

5. Adapted Exercise Programs:

   - Adapting exercise programs to individual abilities and preferences is crucial. Activities like swimming, yoga, and tai chi, which focus on flexibility and balance, can be well-suited for individuals with MS.

6. Rehabilitation Services:
  - Physical and occupational therapy can provide tailored exercise programs and strategies to manage specific mobility challenges. Rehabilitation services play a vital role in optimizing function and independence.

Individuals with MS should work closely with healthcare professionals to develop personalized exercise plans. The goal is to strike a balance that addresses physical capabilities, symptom management, and overall well-being. Regular assessment and adaptation of exercise routines ensure that individuals with MS can derive maximum benefit from physical activity while minimizing potential risks.

Stress Management

Effective stress management is crucial for individuals with Multiple Sclerosis (MS) as stress can exacerbate symptoms and contribute to the overall impact of the condition. Implementing strategies to cope with and reduce stress can significantly enhance the well-being and quality of life for those living with MS.

1. Mindfulness and Meditation:

- Mindfulness practices, including meditation and deep breathing exercises, can help individuals manage stress by promoting relaxation and reducing anxiety. These practices enhance emotional resilience and improve overall mental well-being.

2. Physical Activity:

- Regular exercise not only contributes to physical health but also acts as a powerful stress reducer. Engaging in activities like walking, yoga, or gentle stretching can alleviate tension and promote a sense of calm.

3. Time Management:

- Efficient time management strategies can reduce feelings of overwhelm. Prioritizing tasks, setting realistic goals, and allowing time for breaks contribute to a more manageable daily routine.

4. Social Support:

- Maintaining strong social connections and seeking support from friends, family, or support groups can provide emotional support during challenging times. Sharing experiences and feelings can be therapeutic.

5. Counseling and Psychotherapy:

- Professional counseling or psychotherapy can offer valuable tools for stress management. Cognitive-behavioral therapy, in particular, helps individuals develop coping strategies and resilience in the face of stressors.

6. Healthy Lifestyle Choices:
   - Adopting a healthy lifestyle, including a balanced diet, sufficient sleep, and limiting alcohol and caffeine intake, contributes to overall stress reduction and supports better overall health.

Recognizing the individual nature of stressors and coping mechanisms, individuals with MS may benefit from a combination of these strategies tailored to their unique circumstances. Proactive stress management not only improves the immediate emotional well-being of individuals with MS but may also positively influence the course of the disease by minimizing the impact of stress on symptom exacerbation.

CHAPTER SEVEN

Nutrition and Multiple sclerosis

Nutrition plays a vital role in managing Multiple Sclerosis (MS), contributing to overall health and potentially influencing the course of the disease. While no specific diet can cure MS, adopting a balanced and nutrient-rich eating plan may have beneficial effects on symptom management and well-being.

1. Anti-Inflammatory Foods:
  - An anti-inflammatory diet, rich in fruits, vegetables, whole grains, and healthy fats like those found in fish and nuts, may help modulate inflammation, which is a key factor in MS progression.

2. Omega-3 Fatty Acids:
  - Foods rich in omega-3 fatty acids, such as fatty fish (salmon, mackerel), flaxseeds, and walnuts, may have anti-inflammatory properties that could be beneficial for individuals with MS.

3. Vitamin D:
   - Adequate levels of vitamin D are crucial for individuals with MS, as this vitamin has been associated with a reduced risk of developing the disease and may play a role in its progression. Foods like fatty fish, fortified dairy products, and exposure to sunlight contribute to vitamin D intake.

4. Limiting Saturated Fats:
   - Some studies suggest that reducing the intake of saturated fats, commonly found in red meat and full-fat dairy products, may be beneficial in managing MS symptoms.

5. Hydration:
   - Staying well-hydrated is essential, especially as MS symptoms can be sensitive to dehydration. Opting for water and limiting the intake of sugary beverages supports overall health.

Individuals with MS should work closely with healthcare professionals and registered dietitians to develop personalized nutrition plans. These plans consider individual health needs, dietary preferences, and potential interactions with medications, ensuring a comprehensive and tailored approach to nutrition in the context of Multiple Sclerosis.

The Role of Nutrition

The role of nutrition in the context of Multiple Sclerosis (MS) extends beyond mere sustenance, playing a crucial role in managing symptoms, supporting overall health, and potentially influencing the course of the disease. While no specific diet can cure MS, adopting a well-balanced and individualized approach to nutrition is integral to the holistic management of this chronic neurological condition.

1. Inflammation Modulation:
   - Nutrition can influence inflammation, a key factor in MS progression. An anti-inflammatory diet, rich in fruits, vegetables, whole grains, and omega-3 fatty acids, may help modulate the inflammatory response and potentially alleviate symptoms.

2. Vitamin D Intake:
   - Adequate levels of vitamin D are essential for individuals with MS. Foods rich in vitamin D, such as fatty fish, fortified dairy products, and exposure to sunlight, contribute to overall health and may play a role in disease management.

3. Neuroprotective Nutrients:

- Certain nutrients, including antioxidants and polyphenols found in colorful fruits and vegetables, may have neuroprotective properties. These components potentially contribute to maintaining the health of nerve cells in the central nervous system.

4. Gut Microbiome Influence:

- Emerging research suggests a link between the gut microbiome and MS. A diet that supports a healthy balance of gut bacteria, including the consumption of fiber-rich foods, may positively impact both gut health and overall well-being.

5. Individualized Approaches:

- Recognizing the unique nature of MS and individual responses to dietary interventions, personalized nutrition plans are crucial. Collaboration with healthcare professionals, including dietitians, ensures that nutritional choices align with individual health goals and complement overall MS management strategies.

Understanding the nuanced relationship between nutrition and MS empowers individuals to make informed dietary choices that optimize health and well-being. Integrating nutrition into the comprehensive management of MS supports a holistic approach to living with this complex condition.

A Well-Balanced Diet

A well-balanced diet is the cornerstone of optimal health and is especially crucial for individuals managing conditions such as Multiple Sclerosis (MS). Such a diet provides the necessary nutrients to support overall well-being, mitigate symptoms, and potentially influence the course of chronic conditions.

1. Fruits and Vegetables:
  - Rich in vitamins, minerals, and antioxidants, fruits and vegetables form the foundation of a well-balanced diet. These nutrients contribute to immune function, combat inflammation, and support overall health.

2. Whole Grains:
  - Whole grains, such as brown rice, quinoa, and whole wheat, are excellent sources of fiber, providing sustained energy and promoting digestive health. Fiber also plays a role in managing weight and cholesterol levels.

3. Lean Proteins:
  - Lean protein sources, including poultry, fish, tofu, and legumes, are essential for muscle maintenance, immune function, and overall cellular health. These proteins offer

a nutrient-rich alternative to sources high in saturated fats.

4. Healthy Fats:
   - Incorporating healthy fats, such as those found in avocados, nuts, and olive oil, supports brain health, aids in the absorption of fat-soluble vitamins, and contributes to cardiovascular health.

5. Dairy or Dairy Alternatives:
   - Dairy products or fortified dairy alternatives provide essential nutrients like calcium and vitamin D, crucial for bone health. These nutrients are particularly important for individuals with MS.

6. Hydration:
   - Water is a fundamental component of a well-balanced diet. Staying adequately hydrated supports digestion, helps regulate body temperature, and aids in nutrient transportation.

A well-balanced diet is not only a tool for managing specific health conditions but is a fundamental aspect of preventive healthcare. Tailoring dietary choices to individual needs, considering any specific health conditions, and seeking guidance from healthcare professionals or registered dietitians ensures that individuals can derive maximum benefit from the nutritional components essential for overall health and well-being.

Dietary Considerations

Dietary considerations for individuals with Multiple Sclerosis (MS) go beyond general nutrition, aiming to address specific needs and potential influences on symptom management. While there is no one-size-fits-all approach, several key dietary considerations can play a role in supporting overall health for those living with MS.

1. Anti-Inflammatory Foods:
   - Emphasizing anti-inflammatory foods, including fruits, vegetables, and fatty fish rich in omega-3 fatty acids, may help modulate inflammation and potentially alleviate symptoms associated with MS.

2. Vitamin D Intake:
   - Ensuring adequate vitamin D intake is crucial for individuals with MS, as this vitamin plays a role in immune function and may influence the course of the disease. Foods like fatty fish, fortified dairy, and supplements can contribute to maintaining optimal levels.

3. Balanced Macronutrients:

- Maintaining a balance of macronutrients, including carbohydrates, proteins, and healthy fats, supports overall health and energy levels. This balance is particularly important for individuals managing MS-related fatigue.

4. Hydration:

- Staying well-hydrated is essential, as dehydration can exacerbate symptoms such as fatigue and heat sensitivity. Opting for water and limiting the intake of sugary beverages supports overall health.

5. Individualized Approaches:

- Recognizing the diverse responses to dietary interventions, individualized approaches are key. Collaborating with healthcare professionals, including registered dietitians, ensures that dietary considerations align with individual health goals, preferences, and potential interactions with medications.

By integrating these dietary considerations into an overall management strategy, individuals with MS can optimize nutrition to support their unique health needs and enhance their overall well-being. Regular communication with healthcare providers helps tailor dietary choices to individual circumstances, contributing to a holistic approach to living with MS.

CHAPTER EIGHT

Specific Diets

Several specific diets have been explored in the context of Multiple Sclerosis (MS), aiming to manage symptoms and potentially influence the course of the disease. While research is ongoing, some diets have gained attention for their potential impact on inflammation, immune function, and overall well-being in individuals with MS.

1. Mediterranean Diet:
  - The Mediterranean diet, rich in fruits, vegetables, whole grains, olive oil, and fish, has been associated with anti-inflammatory and neuroprotective effects. Some studies suggest that this diet may contribute to better outcomes for individuals with MS.

2. Low-Fat Diet:
  - A low-fat diet, specifically limiting saturated fats, has been explored due to its potential to reduce

inflammation. Some evidence suggests that reducing the intake of saturated fats from sources like red meat and full-fat dairy may be beneficial for individuals with MS.

3. Gluten-Free Diet:
   - Some individuals with MS choose a gluten-free diet, speculating that it may alleviate symptoms. However, research supporting the widespread adoption of a gluten-free diet for MS management is limited, and its efficacy varies among individuals.

4. Swank Diet:
   - The Swank diet, developed by Dr. Roy Swank, emphasizes low saturated fat intake and high consumption of fish oil. While some early studies suggested benefits, more rigorous research is needed to establish its efficacy in managing MS.

5. Paleolithic Diet:
   - The Paleolithic or "Paleo" diet, which focuses on whole foods and eliminates processed foods, grains, and dairy, has been explored by some individuals with MS. However, evidence supporting its effectiveness in MS management is limited.

It's essential for individuals considering specific diets to consult with healthcare professionals, including registered dietitians, to ensure that dietary choices align with individual health needs and are integrated into a comprehensive MS management plan. Personalized approaches, considering individual responses and preferences, are crucial for optimizing the potential benefits of specific diets in the context of MS.

Mediterranean Diet

The Mediterranean Diet, renowned for its health benefits, has gained attention in the context of managing conditions like Multiple Sclerosis (MS). This dietary pattern, inspired by traditional eating habits in countries bordering the Mediterranean Sea, emphasizes whole, nutrient-rich foods and has been associated with various positive health outcomes.

Central components of the Mediterranean Diet include:

1. Abundant Plant-Based Foods:
   - Fruits, vegetables, whole grains, nuts, and legumes form the foundation, providing essential vitamins, minerals, and fiber.

2. Healthy Fats:
   - Olive oil, a primary source of monounsaturated fats, is a staple. These fats contribute to heart health and may have anti-inflammatory effects.

3. Lean Proteins:

- Fish and poultry are preferred over red meat, offering lean protein and omega-3 fatty acids, potentially influencing inflammation.

4. Moderate Dairy:

- Moderate consumption of dairy, mainly in the form of yogurt and cheese, provides calcium and probiotics.

5. Herbs and Spices:

- Herbs and spices, like basil, oregano, and garlic, add flavor without relying on excessive salt, promoting overall cardiovascular health.

6. Occasional Red Wine:

- Red wine, consumed in moderation and often with meals, has been associated with antioxidant properties and heart health.

Research suggests that the Mediterranean Diet's emphasis on anti-inflammatory and neuroprotective components may have potential benefits for individuals with MS. While not a cure, adopting this dietary pattern, coupled with personalized considerations and healthcare guidance, may contribute to overall well-being for those managing MS.

Low-Fat Diets

Low-fat diets have been explored for their potential health benefits, including in the context of managing conditions like Multiple Sclerosis (MS). These dietary patterns focus on reducing the intake of saturated fats, which are commonly found in animal products, processed foods, and certain cooking oils. While research on the direct impact of low-fat diets on MS is ongoing, some individuals adopt these dietary approaches for potential anti-inflammatory effects and cardiovascular benefits.

Key components of low-fat diets include:

1. Lean Proteins:
   - Emphasis is placed on lean protein sources such as poultry, fish, beans, and legumes, reducing the intake of saturated fats commonly found in red meat.

2. Plant-Based Fats:
   - Healthy fats from plant sources, such as avocados, nuts, and olive oil, are often included. These fats provide essential fatty acids and may have anti-inflammatory properties.

3. Whole Grains:

- Whole grains, rich in fiber and nutrients, are a staple. They contribute to sustained energy and support digestive health.

4. Limiting Saturated Fats:
- Processed foods, fried foods, and certain oils high in saturated fats are limited to promote heart health and potentially modulate inflammation.

While the evidence supporting low-fat diets in MS management is not conclusive, some studies suggest potential benefits in reducing inflammation. However, the individualized nature of dietary responses emphasizes the importance of consulting with healthcare professionals, including registered dietitians, to ensure that dietary choices align with overall health goals and complement comprehensive MS management strategies.

High-Vitamin D Diets

High-vitamin D diets have garnered attention, particularly in the context of conditions like Multiple Sclerosis (MS), where vitamin D is believed to play a crucial role. Vitamin D is essential for immune function, and deficiency has been associated with an increased risk of developing MS and potentially influencing disease progression.

Key components of high-vitamin D diets include:

1. Fatty Fish:
   - Fatty fish such as salmon, mackerel, and trout are excellent sources of vitamin D. Regular consumption can contribute to maintaining optimal vitamin D levels.

2. Fortified Foods:
   - Fortified dairy products, plant-based milk alternatives, and cereals often contain added vitamin D, providing options for individuals with dietary restrictions or limited sun exposure.

3. Egg Yolks:
   - Egg yolks are a natural source of vitamin D and can be incorporated into various dishes as part of a high-vitamin D diet.

4. Mushrooms:
   - Certain types of mushrooms, when exposed to sunlight or ultraviolet (UV) light during growth, naturally accumulate vitamin D. Including these mushrooms in the diet adds a plant-based source of vitamin D.

5. Supplements:
   - In some cases, vitamin D supplements may be recommended to ensure adequate intake, especially for individuals with limited sun exposure.

While maintaining sufficient vitamin D levels is essential, it's crucial to approach dietary choices as part of a comprehensive MS management plan. Consultation with healthcare professionals, including registered dietitians, helps tailor dietary strategies to individual needs, ensuring that high-vitamin D diets align with overall health goals for those managing MS.

Controversies and Considerations

The management of Multiple Sclerosis (MS) is complex, and various controversies and considerations surround its dietary aspects. It's essential for individuals with MS to approach dietary choices with careful consideration and awareness of ongoing research. Here are key points to navigate these complexities:

1. Controversial Diets:
   - Some specific diets, such as the Swank diet, gluten-free diet, or paleolithic diet, have been proposed as potential strategies for managing MS. However, the evidence supporting their widespread adoption remains inconclusive, and the efficacy may vary among individuals.

2. Individual Responses:
   - Responses to dietary interventions can be highly individualized. What works for one person may not work for another. It's crucial to consider individual health

needs, preferences, and tolerances when exploring dietary choices.

3. Professional Guidance:
   - Consultation with healthcare professionals, including neurologists and registered dietitians, is paramount. These experts can provide personalized advice, considering the individual's overall health, specific symptoms, and potential interactions with medications.

4. Balanced Nutrition:
   - While certain diets may be explored, maintaining a well-balanced and nutrient-rich diet remains a fundamental principle. A balanced diet ensures the intake of essential nutrients needed for overall health and well-being.

5. Research and Evolving Understanding:
   - The field of nutritional research in MS is continually evolving. Staying informed about the latest research findings and being open to adjustments in dietary strategies based on emerging evidence is crucial.

Navigating the controversies and considerations related to diet and MS requires a nuanced and individualized approach. Informed decision-making, professional guidance, and a commitment to overall well-being contribute to a holistic strategy for individuals managing the complexities of Multiple Sclerosis.

CHAPTER NINE

Supplements

Supplements play a role in the management of Multiple Sclerosis (MS), complementing dietary strategies to address potential nutrient deficiencies and support overall health. While individual needs may vary, several supplements are commonly considered:

1. Vitamin D:
   - Vitamin D is crucial for individuals with MS, and supplements may be recommended, especially for those with limited sun exposure. Maintaining optimal vitamin D levels is associated with potential benefits in disease management.

2. Omega-3 Fatty Acids:
   - Omega-3 supplements, often derived from fish oil, provide essential fatty acids with potential anti-inflammatory properties. These supplements are

explored for their impact on MS symptoms and disease progression.

3. B Vitamins:
  - B vitamins, including B12 and B9 (folate), are important for neurological health. Individuals with MS, especially those on certain medications, may consider supplements to ensure adequate intake.

4. Calcium and Vitamin K:
  - Maintaining bone health is crucial for individuals with MS, and supplements of calcium and vitamin K may be recommended, particularly if dairy intake is limited.

5. Iron:
  - Iron supplements may be considered for individuals with MS who are at risk of anemia, which can contribute to fatigue.

It's crucial to approach supplements under the guidance of healthcare professionals, considering individual health needs and potential interactions with medications. Regular monitoring and adjustments ensure that supplement regimens align with overall MS management plans, contributing to the holistic well-being of individuals navigating the complexities of this neurological condition.

Vitamin D and MS

The relationship between Vitamin D and Multiple Sclerosis (MS) has been a subject of considerable research, highlighting the potential significance of this essential vitamin in both the development and management of the disease. Vitamin D, known for its role in calcium absorption and bone health, has garnered attention for its immunomodulatory properties, impacting the immune system and potentially influencing the inflammatory processes associated with MS.

Research suggests several key points regarding Vitamin D and MS:

1. Association with Risk:

 - There is evidence to suggest that individuals with lower Vitamin D levels may have an increased risk of developing MS. Sunlight exposure, diet, and supplements contribute to Vitamin D status.

2. Potential Impact on Disease Progression:

 - Adequate Vitamin D levels may be associated with a reduced risk of relapses and slower progression of disability in individuals with MS.

3. Immunomodulatory Effects:

- Vitamin D plays a role in regulating immune responses, and deficiency may contribute to dysregulation. Modulating the immune system is of particular interest in managing autoimmune conditions like MS.

4. Supplementation Considerations:

- Vitamin D supplementation is commonly recommended for individuals with MS, especially in regions with limited sunlight. Healthcare professionals often monitor Vitamin D levels and adjust supplementation as needed.

While the relationship between Vitamin D and MS is complex and not fully understood, maintaining optimal Vitamin D levels through a combination of sunlight exposure, dietary sources, and supplements may contribute to overall well-being and potentially impact the course of the disease. Individualized approaches, considering factors like geographic location and lifestyle, are crucial when addressing Vitamin D in the context of MS.

Omega-3 Fatty Acids

Omega-3 fatty acids are essential polyunsaturated fats that play a crucial role in maintaining overall health, and their potential benefits have been explored in the context of conditions like Multiple Sclerosis (MS). These fatty acids, primarily found in certain fish, flaxseeds, chia seeds, and walnuts, consist of three main types: alpha-linolenic acid (ALA), eicosapentaenoic acid (EPA), and docosahexaenoic acid (DHA).

Research suggests several key points regarding Omega-3 fatty acids and MS:

1. Anti-Inflammatory Properties:
   - Omega-3 fatty acids are known for their anti-inflammatory properties. In the context of MS, where inflammation contributes to disease progression, these fats may have potential benefits in modulating the immune response.

2. Potential Impact on Symptoms:
   - Some studies have explored the impact of Omega-3 fatty acids on MS symptoms, particularly in relation to fatigue and cognitive function. While evidence is not

conclusive, there is interest in their role in managing certain aspects of the condition.

3. Sources and Supplementation:
   - Fatty fish like salmon, mackerel, and sardines are rich sources of EPA and DHA. For individuals with dietary restrictions or preferences, supplements such as fish oil capsules or algae-based supplements can provide Omega-3 fatty acids.

While Omega-3 fatty acids are recognized for their potential health benefits, individual responses may vary. Consulting with healthcare professionals, including neurologists and dietitians, ensures that incorporating these fats into the diet aligns with overall health goals and complements comprehensive strategies for managing MS.

Consultation with Healthcare Professionals

Consultation with healthcare professionals is a fundamental aspect of managing Multiple Sclerosis (MS), ensuring that individuals receive personalized and comprehensive care tailored to their unique needs. Neurologists, registered dietitians, and other specialists play critical roles in guiding individuals through the complexities of MS management.

1. Neurologists:

- Neurologists specialize in the nervous system and are central to the diagnosis and ongoing management of MS. They prescribe medications, monitor disease progression, and provide guidance on symptom management.

2. Registered Dietitians:

- Dietitians offer expert advice on nutrition, helping individuals with MS make informed dietary choices. They consider factors like potential interactions with medications, address specific symptoms, and create personalized nutrition plans.

3. Rehabilitation Specialists:

- Physical and occupational therapists assist individuals in maintaining or improving mobility, managing fatigue, and addressing specific challenges associated with MS. Rehabilitation services play a vital role in enhancing overall function and independence.

4. Mental Health Professionals:

- Psychologists or counselors help individuals navigate the emotional and psychological aspects of living with a chronic condition. Managing stress, anxiety, and depression is integral to comprehensive MS care.

5. Primary Care Physicians:
   - Primary care physicians coordinate overall healthcare and may address general health concerns. Regular check-ups with primary care providers contribute to holistic health management.

Consultation with healthcare professionals ensures a collaborative and multidisciplinary approach to MS care. Regular communication allows for adjustments in treatment plans, addressing emerging symptoms, and optimizing overall well-being. Individuals with MS and their healthcare teams work together to develop strategies that align with personal health goals, fostering a proactive and individualized approach to managing this complex condition.

CHAPTER TEN

Preventive Measures

Preventive measures are crucial for individuals seeking to manage and potentially reduce the risk of developing Multiple Sclerosis (MS), a complex neurological condition. While the exact cause of MS remains unknown, several lifestyle and health strategies may contribute to overall well-being and possibly impact disease outcomes.

1. Maintaining a Healthy Lifestyle:
   - Adopting a well-balanced diet, engaging in regular physical activity, managing stress, and avoiding tobacco use contribute to overall health. These lifestyle factors are linked to better immune function and may play a role in reducing the risk of MS.

2. Adequate Vitamin D Intake:

- Ensuring sufficient vitamin D levels through sunlight exposure, diet, and supplements, if necessary, is associated with a potential reduction in MS risk and may positively influence disease progression.

3. Regular Exercise:
- Engaging in regular physical activity supports cardiovascular health, reduces the risk of obesity, and may have positive effects on the immune system. Exercise is also associated with improved mood and cognitive function.

4. Mindfulness and Stress Management:
- Practices such as mindfulness, meditation, and stress management techniques contribute to emotional well-being. Chronic stress has been linked to immune dysregulation and may influence MS susceptibility and progression.

5. Regular Health Check-ups:
- Periodic health check-ups with primary care providers facilitate the early detection and management of health conditions, contributing to overall preventive care.

While no guaranteed preventive measures exist for MS, adopting a proactive and health-conscious lifestyle can positively impact general well-being and potentially influence the complex interplay of factors contributing to the development and progression of MS. Consultation with healthcare professionals can provide personalized guidance on preventive strategies based on individual health profiles.

Lifestyle Choices

Lifestyle choices significantly influence the well-being of individuals, and for those managing or seeking to prevent conditions like Multiple Sclerosis (MS), thoughtful decisions regarding various aspects of life can have a profound impact. Several key lifestyle choices contribute to overall health and may play a role in managing MS:

1. Nutrition:
   - Adopting a balanced and nutrient-rich diet, emphasizing fruits, vegetables, whole grains, and lean proteins, provides essential nutrients and supports overall health. For individuals with MS, dietary choices may also include considerations for potential anti-inflammatory effects.

2. Physical Activity:
   - Regular exercise is crucial for cardiovascular health, weight management, and maintaining mobility. Tailored exercise regimens, taking into account individual

capabilities and symptoms, contribute to overall well-being for those with MS.

3. Stress Management:
   - Implementing stress-reducing strategies, such as mindfulness, meditation, or engaging in hobbies, is essential. Chronic stress can impact MS symptoms, and effective stress management is integral to holistic care.

4. Sleep Hygiene:
   - Prioritizing sufficient and quality sleep is vital for overall health. Sleep disturbances are common in MS, and establishing good sleep hygiene practices can contribute to better symptom management.

5. Avoidance of Tobacco and Limiting Alcohol:
   - Avoiding tobacco use and limiting alcohol intake are key lifestyle choices that support overall health. These habits contribute to cardiovascular health and reduce the risk of certain MS-related complications.

Making informed lifestyle choices empowers individuals to take an active role in their health. Consulting with healthcare professionals, including neurologists and lifestyle specialists, ensures that lifestyle choices align with overall health goals and contribute to a comprehensive approach to managing and preventing health conditions such as MS.

Emerging Research on Prevention

Emerging research on the prevention of Multiple Sclerosis (MS) is shedding light on potential strategies to reduce the risk of developing this complex neurological condition. While the exact cause of MS remains elusive, ongoing investigations are exploring various factors that may contribute to prevention.

1. Early-Life Exposures:
   - Studies suggest that exposures and experiences during early life, such as infections, diet, and environmental factors, may influence the risk of developing MS. Understanding these early-life factors is a key focus in preventive research.

2. Microbiome and Gut Health:
   - The role of the gut microbiome in immune regulation is a burgeoning area of research. Emerging evidence suggests that a balanced and diverse gut microbiome may contribute to a healthier immune system, potentially impacting MS risk.

3. Vitamin D and Sunlight Exposure:
   - Vitamin D deficiency has been linked to an increased risk of MS. Research is exploring the impact of

optimizing vitamin D levels through sunlight exposure or supplementation as a preventive measure.

4. Immunomodulation:
  - Investigating ways to modulate the immune system early in life is a focus of preventive research. This includes understanding how exposures to various pathogens and vaccinations may shape immune responses and potentially influence MS risk.

5. Genetic Factors:
  - Ongoing genetic research aims to identify specific genetic factors that may contribute to susceptibility or resilience to MS. Understanding the interplay between genetic and environmental factors is crucial for developing targeted preventive strategies.

As research continues to uncover new insights, preventive measures may evolve, offering hope for reducing the incidence and impact of MS. Individuals at risk or with a family history of MS may benefit from staying informed about emerging research findings and consulting with healthcare professionals for personalized guidance on preventive measures.

CHAPTER ELEVEN

Research and Future Therapies

Research on Multiple Sclerosis (MS) is dynamic and holds promise for future therapies that could revolutionize the management and treatment of this complex neurological condition. Scientists are exploring diverse avenues, focusing on both symptom management and disease modification.

1. Immunomodulation and Immune Therapies:
   - Advances in immunomodulation aim to regulate the immune system's response, potentially slowing down disease progression. Immune therapies, including monoclonal antibodies and other targeted approaches, are under investigation for their efficacy in modifying the course of MS.

2. Neuroprotective Strategies:

- Research is focused on identifying compounds and interventions that protect nerve cells in the central nervous system, with the goal of preserving function and potentially repairing damage caused by MS.

3. Myelin Repair and Regeneration:
- Strategies to stimulate myelin repair and regeneration are a critical focus. Researchers are exploring ways to promote the restoration of myelin, the protective covering of nerve fibers damaged in MS.

4. Precision Medicine:
- Advancements in understanding the genetic and molecular factors contributing to MS are paving the way for precision medicine approaches. Tailoring treatments based on individual characteristics may enhance effectiveness and reduce side effects.

5. Emerging Technologies:
- Technologies such as advanced imaging, biomarker identification, and artificial intelligence are accelerating research. These tools provide insights into disease mechanisms, aiding in the development of more targeted and personalized therapeutic strategies.

As research progresses, the landscape of MS treatment is expected to evolve, offering new hope for improved outcomes and quality of life for individuals living with this condition. Continued support for research initiatives, clinical trials, and collaboration among scientists and healthcare professionals is crucial for bringing these future therapies to fruition.

Ongoing Research

Ongoing research on Multiple Sclerosis (MS) is advancing our understanding of the disease and shaping innovative approaches to treatment and management. Current investigations span various areas, contributing to a more nuanced comprehension of the complex interplay of genetic, environmental, and immune factors in MS.

1. Genomic Studies:
   - Researchers are delving into the genetic basis of MS, identifying specific genetic markers associated with susceptibility and disease progression. These studies aim to unravel the intricate genetic landscape of MS and provide insights into potential therapeutic targets.

2. Immunological Mechanisms:
   - Ongoing research explores the immune system's role in MS, investigating factors that contribute to immune dysregulation and the subsequent attack on the central nervous system. Understanding these mechanisms is

crucial for developing targeted immunomodulatory therapies.

3. Biomarkers and Imaging:
- Advances in biomarker identification and imaging technologies are enhancing diagnostic accuracy and providing insights into disease activity. Biomarkers offer potential indicators for disease progression and treatment response.

4. Neuroprotection and Repair:
- Researchers are focusing on strategies for neuroprotection and myelin repair, aiming to preserve and restore nerve function. This area of research holds promise for developing therapies that go beyond symptom management to address the underlying damage caused by MS.

5. Environmental Triggers:
- Investigations into environmental factors, such as viral infections and lifestyle influences, aim to identify triggers that may contribute to the onset and progression of MS. Understanding these factors can inform preventive strategies and lifestyle recommendations.

Ongoing research initiatives are dynamic, with the potential to uncover groundbreaking insights that may lead to more effective treatments and improved outcomes for individuals with MS. The collaborative efforts of scientists, clinicians, and individuals living with MS are essential for advancing knowledge and translating discoveries into tangible benefits for those affected by this challenging condition.

Emerging Therapies

Emerging therapies for Multiple Sclerosis (MS) represent a frontier in neurological research, offering new avenues for improved symptom management and potentially disease modification. These innovative approaches span various strategies, reflecting a nuanced understanding of the complex mechanisms underlying MS.

1. B-cell Targeted Therapies:
   - B cells, a type of immune cell, are implicated in MS pathology. Emerging therapies specifically target these cells to modulate the immune response and reduce inflammation, potentially slowing down disease progression.

2. Stem Cell Therapies:
   - Stem cell research holds promise for MS treatment by aiming to repair damaged myelin and regenerate nerve cells. Clinical trials exploring the transplantation of stem

cells seek to harness their regenerative potential for neurological recovery.

3. Neuroprotective Agents:
   - Novel neuroprotective agents are under investigation to shield nerve cells from damage and enhance their survival. These therapies target mechanisms involved in the protection of neurons, potentially preserving function in the central nervous system.

4. Remylination Strategies:
   - Therapies designed to stimulate remyelination, the process of rebuilding the protective myelin sheath around nerve fibers, are actively being explored. These approaches aim to address one of the key aspects of MS pathology and promote functional recovery.

5. Precision Medicine Approaches:
   - Advances in understanding the individualized nature of MS are leading to precision medicine approaches. Tailoring treatments based on genetic, molecular, and clinical characteristics may enhance efficacy and minimize side effects.

While many of these therapies are in the early stages of research or clinical trials, they offer hope for a future where MS management goes beyond symptom control to address the underlying mechanisms of the disease, potentially transforming the outlook for individuals living with MS. Continued support for research initiatives and collaboration between scientists, healthcare professionals, and individuals affected by MS are crucial for bringing these emerging therapies to fruition.

Hope for the Future

The future of Multiple Sclerosis (MS) holds promise as ongoing research, and emerging therapies open new avenues for understanding, managing, and potentially preventing this complex neurological condition. Several factors inspire hope for individuals affected by MS:

1. Advancements in Understanding:
   - The depth of research into the genetic, environmental, and immunological aspects of MS continues to expand. A more nuanced understanding of the disease mechanisms provides a solid foundation for developing targeted therapies.

2. Precision Medicine:
   - The shift toward precision medicine is tailoring treatments based on individual characteristics. This personalized approach recognizes the unique nature of MS, allowing for more effective and individualized strategies.

3. Neuroprotective and Remyelination Therapies:
   - Emerging therapies targeting neuroprotection and remyelination aim to address the underlying damage caused by MS. If successful, these approaches could revolutionize the treatment landscape by promoting healing and functional recovery.

4. B-cell and Immune Therapies:
   - Innovative therapies targeting B cells and modulating the immune response show promise in managing inflammation and slowing disease progression. These approaches offer hope for improved symptom control and potentially halting the advancement of MS.

5. Stem Cell Research:
   - Stem cell research holds tremendous potential for repairing damaged nerves and promoting regeneration. Clinical trials exploring stem cell transplantation offer a glimpse into future possibilities for neurological recovery.

While challenges persist, the collaborative efforts of researchers, healthcare professionals, individuals living with MS, and advocacy groups fuel the optimism for a future where the management of MS is not only more effective but also tailored to the unique needs of each individual. The pursuit of breakthroughs and the commitment to advancing knowledge inspire hope for a future where the impact of MS is significantly mitigated.

CHAPTER TWELVE

Support Networks

Support networks play a crucial role in the lives of individuals affected by Multiple Sclerosis (MS), providing emotional, practical, and informational assistance that is vital for navigating the challenges associated with this complex condition. These networks encompass a variety of sources:

1. Family and Friends:
   - Close relationships with family and friends form the bedrock of support. Emotional understanding, companionship, and assistance with daily tasks contribute to the overall well-being of individuals with MS.

2. Peer Support Groups:
   - Connecting with others who share similar experiences through peer support groups offers a sense of community and understanding. Shared insights,

coping strategies, and empathy create a supportive environment for individuals with MS.

3. Healthcare Professionals:
   - Collaborating with a multidisciplinary healthcare team, including neurologists, physical therapists, and mental health professionals, ensures comprehensive care. Regular communication with healthcare providers helps address evolving needs and adjust management strategies.

4. Online Communities:
   - Virtual platforms and online communities provide a space for individuals with MS to share information, seek advice, and find encouragement. These communities foster a sense of belonging and offer valuable insights from diverse perspectives.

5. Advocacy Organizations:
   - Organizations dedicated to MS advocacy and awareness offer resources, education, and opportunities for advocacy. These groups empower individuals to navigate healthcare systems, access information, and contribute to the broader MS community.

Building and maintaining a robust support network is essential for enhancing resilience and quality of life for individuals with MS. The combined strength of these supportive relationships creates a foundation that helps individuals face the challenges of MS with greater confidence and optimism.

Importance of Support

The importance of support in the context of Multiple Sclerosis (MS) cannot be overstated, as it plays a pivotal role in the physical, emotional, and social well-being of individuals navigating this complex neurological condition.

1. Emotional Well-being:
   - Living with a chronic condition like MS can evoke a range of emotions, including fear, frustration, and anxiety. A strong support system, comprised of family, friends, and peers, provides a safe space to express these emotions, fostering emotional resilience and mental well-being.

2. Practical Assistance:
   - The daily challenges associated with MS, such as mobility issues or fatigue, often necessitate practical support. Whether it's help with household tasks, transportation, or personal care, a supportive network lightens the burden and enhances the individual's quality of life.

3. Information and Education:

- Support networks offer access to valuable information and resources related to MS. From treatment options to lifestyle strategies, being well-informed empowers individuals to make educated decisions about their health and management strategies.

4. Reducing Social Isolation:

- MS can sometimes lead to social isolation due to physical limitations or misconceptions about the condition. Supportive relationships combat isolation, providing companionship and fostering a sense of belonging within the broader community.

5. Advocacy and Empowerment:

- Support networks, including advocacy organizations, empower individuals with MS to be advocates for themselves. Through shared experiences and collective efforts, individuals can raise awareness, influence policy, and contribute to a more supportive and inclusive environment.

In essence, the importance of support lies in its transformative impact on the overall quality of life for individuals with MS. It not only addresses the practical challenges of managing the condition but also contributes significantly to emotional resilience, empowerment, and a sense of connectedness within a larger, understanding community.

Community Resources

Community resources are invaluable for individuals affected by Multiple Sclerosis (MS), providing a range of support services, information, and assistance tailored to the unique needs of those navigating this neurological condition.

1. MS Support Groups:
  - Local and online MS support groups offer a platform for individuals to connect, share experiences, and exchange practical advice. These groups foster a sense of community, understanding, and mutual support.

2. Rehabilitation Centers:
  - Rehabilitation centers specializing in neurological conditions, including MS, provide access to physical therapy, occupational therapy, and other rehabilitative services. These centers play a crucial role in enhancing mobility, managing symptoms, and improving overall function.

3. Patient Education Programs:
  - Educational programs organized by community resources offer individuals and their families valuable information about MS. These programs cover various

aspects, including disease management, treatment options, and strategies for coping with specific symptoms.

4. Transportation Services:

- Many communities provide transportation services for individuals with mobility challenges, ensuring accessibility to medical appointments, support group meetings, and other essential activities.

5. Home Healthcare Services:

- Community-based home healthcare services offer assistance with daily activities, enabling individuals with MS to maintain independence while receiving necessary support in the comfort of their homes.

6. Assistive Technology Programs:

- Community resources often include programs that provide access to assistive technologies, such as mobility aids or communication devices, tailored to the needs of individuals with MS.

These community resources form a crucial part of the comprehensive support network for individuals with MS, addressing diverse needs and contributing to an inclusive and empowering environment for those managing this complex condition. Accessing and leveraging these resources enhances the overall well-being and quality of life for individuals and their families affected by MS.

Building a Supportive Network

Building a supportive network is essential for individuals navigating the challenges of Multiple Sclerosis (MS), creating a foundation of understanding, encouragement, and practical assistance. Constructing such a network involves intentional efforts and a recognition of the diverse forms of support needed:

1. Open Communication:
   - Fostering open communication with family, friends, and healthcare providers is fundamental. Clearly expressing needs, concerns, and goals promotes mutual understanding and enables others to provide meaningful support.

2. Education and Awareness:
   - Providing information about MS to those in the support network helps demystify the condition. Increased awareness promotes empathy and equips individuals to offer informed and effective support.

3. Involving Family and Friends:

- Involving close relationships in the management of MS encourages a shared responsibility for well-being. Friends and family can contribute to both emotional support and practical assistance.

4. Seeking Peer Connections:

- Connecting with peers who share similar experiences creates a unique bond. Peer support groups or online communities provide a platform for sharing insights, coping strategies, and encouragement.

5. Professional Guidance:

- Involving healthcare professionals, including neurologists and rehabilitation specialists, in the support network ensures comprehensive care. Regular communication with these professionals aids in adapting strategies to evolving needs.

6. Community Resources:

- Leveraging community resources, such as MS support groups, rehabilitation centers, and educational programs, expands the network and provides access to a broader range of assistance and information.

Building a supportive network is a dynamic process that evolves over time. By cultivating strong connections and involving various sources of support, individuals with MS can enhance their resilience and navigate the complexities of the condition with a sense of empowerment and community.

Conclusion

In conclusion, the landscape of Multiple Sclerosis (MS) is evolving, propelled by advancements in research, emerging therapies, and a growing understanding of the complex factors influencing this neurological condition. From the intricacies of its autoimmune nature to the impact on daily life, the narrative of MS is shaped by a diverse array of elements.

While the journey with MS poses formidable challenges, there is a resounding message of hope for the future. Ongoing research and innovative therapies hold the promise of more effective treatments, potentially altering the trajectory of the disease. The importance of support networks, encompassing family, friends, healthcare professionals, and community resources, cannot be overstated. These networks contribute immeasurably to the emotional well-being, practical assistance, and advocacy for those affected by MS.

As individuals with MS and their support systems face the complexities of diagnosis, symptom management, and lifestyle considerations, the emphasis on a multidisciplinary and individualized approach becomes increasingly clear. The integration of medical interventions, lifestyle choices, and a supportive community creates a holistic framework for managing MS.

Ultimately, the journey with MS is marked by resilience, empowerment, and the collaborative efforts of researchers, healthcare professionals, and individuals themselves. In the pursuit of a better understanding, enhanced treatments, and improved quality of life, the collective commitment to unraveling the complexities of MS remains steadfast, offering a beacon of hope for those affected by this condition.

Summary of Key Points

In summary, exploring the intricate landscape of Multiple Sclerosis (MS) reveals key points crucial for understanding, managing, and offering support for individuals affected by this complex neurological condition:

1. Diverse Nature of MS: MS is a multifaceted condition with diverse symptoms, ranging from fatigue and mobility challenges to cognitive impairment. Its autoimmune nature involves the immune system mistakenly attacking the central nervous system.

2. Risk Factors and Demographics: While the exact cause of MS remains unknown, factors such as genetics, environmental triggers, and geographical location contribute to risk. MS often affects individuals in their prime adulthood, with women more commonly affected than men.

3. Types and Progression: MS presents in various forms, including Relapsing-Remitting (RRMS), Secondary Progressive (SPMS), and Primary Progressive (PPMS). The progression of the disease is unpredictable, impacting individuals differently.

4. Diagnosis and Diagnostic Process: Diagnosing MS involves a comprehensive process, including medical examinations, tests, and imaging. Early intervention and accurate diagnosis are crucial for effective management.

5. Impact on Daily Life: MS affects various aspects of daily life, presenting physical, emotional, and social challenges. Coping strategies and a supportive network play essential roles in enhancing the quality of life.

6. Treatment Landscape: Medical treatments, including disease-modifying medications, aim to manage symptoms and slow disease progression. Early intervention is emphasized for optimal outcomes.

7. Lifestyle Factors: Lifestyle choices, including nutrition, exercise, stress management, and adequate sleep, contribute significantly to overall well-being for individuals with MS.

8. Hope for the Future: Emerging research, therapies, and a growing understanding of MS inspire hope for improved treatments, enhanced quality of life, and potential preventive measures.

In conclusion, the journey with MS is multifaceted, emphasizing the importance of a comprehensive, individualized approach that incorporates medical, lifestyle, and supportive components. As research advances and awareness deepens, the collective efforts of individuals, healthcare professionals, and the broader community continue to shape a hopeful future for those impacted by MS.

Encouragement and Empowerment

Encouragement and empowerment are indispensable pillars in the journey of individuals facing Multiple Sclerosis (MS). Navigating the challenges posed by this complex condition requires not only medical interventions but also a resilient mindset and a robust support system.

Encouragement plays a vital role in bolstering the emotional well-being of those with MS. A positive and understanding environment, coupled with empathetic communication from family, friends, and healthcare providers, fosters a sense of optimism. Encouragement helps individuals confront the uncertainties of MS with greater resilience, promoting mental strength and adaptability.

Empowerment goes hand-in-hand with encouragement, providing individuals with the tools and knowledge to actively participate in their healthcare journey. Being informed about treatment options, lifestyle choices, and available support resources empowers individuals to make decisions aligned with their unique needs and preferences. Encouraging self-advocacy and fostering a sense of control over aspects of life, despite the challenges posed by MS, enhances overall well-being.

Moreover, encouragement and empowerment extend beyond the individual to the broader support network. Educating family, friends, and the community about MS cultivates an understanding and inclusive environment, further reinforcing the sense of empowerment for those affected.

In the face of the uncertainties associated with MS, the dual forces of encouragement and empowerment serve as beacons of strength, enabling individuals to navigate their journey with resilience, hope, and a proactive spirit.